IVF and trying to conceive? Been there, done that and this is what you need to know.

JOANNE THORNTON

It's hard waiting around for something you know might never happen, but it's even harder to give up when you know it's everything you want – anonymous

Contents

1.

Beginning

So this is a story about little old me, otherwise known as Mum, Jo or Joanne when I'm in trouble. I'm just a normal everyday person living my life like anyone else.

I'm not special, there are thousands of women out there like me who have gone through or are going through a scary, lonely, painful and emotional ride called the IVF roller coaster. Such highs and then some lows that can be devastating.

The only thing that makes you keep going is the hope that you will finish your journey on that magical high where you are holding ever so tightly that precious bundle of joy.

In saying that there are so many things that you should be aware of before you start IVF or any type of assisted conception. I didn't know enough when I started and wished I had so hopefully my story will make you better prepared for your journey.

If you're already going through this then maybe it will make you feel not quite so alone and hopefully you can take some comfort from knowing that your feelings are believe it or not normal.

If you have someone close to you going through this challenging time you might be able to get a better understanding of what they are living through day by day and hopefully be able to help them or just be there for them.

I have included some notes I made whilst going through some of my cycles. Looking back and reading them I can hear how desperate my words were and how I would cling to anything in the hope that I might have been pregnant. I can also feel the sadness and despair.

I'm hoping that this book can help some of you out there who may be going through a really tough time.

2.

Our Start

You always think you know how life will go. You meet someone, get married and have babies. It should be pretty simple and you never think twice about it happening any other way, but what if it doesn't turn out the way you expect and your dreams don't come true?

From the time I was a little girl you could always find me playing with my dolls (my babies), I had always known I wanted to be a mum.

When I left school I wanted a great job but I didn't want a career. I just wanted to find someone wonderful to marry and then have my babies.

I was lucky enough to meet my husband at a young age and after eight years we were married.

We wanted to wait a little while before starting a family but I received the shock of my life a year later when I found out I had a malignant melanoma. I was extremely lucky that it was caught at stage two so I didn't need to have chemotherapy or any other treatment but if I had left it for a few more months I would have been in a fight for my life and I might never have had the chance to even try for children.

Even though I was okay I had check-ups every three months and I found it quite hard to deal with my own mortality so babies were put on the back burner. I also wanted to make sure that the cancer didn't return so we waited a bit longer.

When we finally started trying to conceive we were so excited, this would be a whole new chapter in our lives. We thought it was going to be easy. After all the majority of my family seem to be extremely fertile so when we weren't pregnant after six months I was surprised.

I decided to consult a doctor who said not to worry as I was still young so I didn't get a referral for a specialist for another few months. She said we would probably fall pregnant before we got an appointment so we tried everything.

I did Ovulation Predictor Kits (which involved peeing on a stick), checking my cervical mucus for the 'right' time, even laying on my back with my legs in the air after intercourse. Looking back now I can laugh thinking of some of these things but I would have done anything.

When I saw the specialist he did lots of different tests and everything seemed fine so he thought it might be something called unexplained infertility.

I ended up having a laparoscopy which showed I had severe endometriosis. My ovaries were stuck down to my uterus so I had all of it removed and even though the recovery was quite painful at least it was all gone and we could start trying again.

Six months later we still weren't pregnant so we decided to try Inter Uterine Insemination (IUI) which thankfully worked on our second cycle.

IUI has some similarities with IVF, you still have to inject yourself with the hormones every day and have numerous blood tests. When the blood tests show you are nearly ready you have an internal ultrasound to see how big your eggs are and how many you have, you then take another injection (it's called a trigger injection) to start the release of your egg or eggs. The final step is to have your partner do a sperm sample. It is cleaned and divided so you only have healthy sperm and then it's inseminated by a catheter which feels a bit like a pap smear.

When we wanted our second baby I again fell pregnant with IUI on our fourth cycle but unfortunately we lost our baby.

It was then another six months of doing IUI with no success and trying to decide whether to do IVF. I was a bit scared of IVF and worried about the cost involved but then something amazing happened, we won some money on a television show.

It seemed like it was meant to be so that made our minds up, we were going to pull out the big guns and try IVF or as I like to call it 'Invasive Vaginal Forensics'. Trust me you have to find humour wherever you can get it!

We fell pregnant on our very first IVF cycle and have five perfect little embryos sitting on ice.

3.
Planning

Looking back on our journey I wish I had been more prepared. You go in to see your doctor and listen to what's going to happen and you think great, we're going to get a baby. Being so focused or one sided about the end result you don't really 'hear' what the doctor is saying.

I think everyone starting IVF or any other type of assisted conception should have counselling or speak to someone who has been there, done that. You need to find out what it is truly going to be like. I was totally overwhelmed by the side effects of the hormones I was injecting and it was extremely difficult for both me and my family to handle.

You also need to know how time consuming this commitment will be. You are regularly having appointments and sometimes you can be phoned late in the afternoon and need to be at the clinic early the next morning which can be difficult if you work or have other children to consider.

Having family or friends that can take your child or children at short notice is a must. My poor daughter was dragged along to all of my blood tests which were enough for her to have to see but most of the other appointments you wouldn't want your children to be there.

You need to discuss, get or sort out how much money you will need for this process. It's hard enough without the financial burden on top of everything else involved.

Plan what lengths you are willing to go to. By this I mean if you aren't able to fall pregnant would you consider donor eggs or donor sperm?

Give yourself a time limit. For example do treatment for a year but then if it hasn't worked take three or four months off from your treatment.

Once you're in that IVF daze it's very difficult to be rational and make the appropriate decisions because you are so caught up in this baby making bubble where you only see one goal, a baby. You end up thinking that a baby is all there is in life and nothing else matters.

The worst thing you can do is lose sight of yourself, your partner and who you are together as a couple. This is so easy to do so if you plan to take those months off between treatments you can reconnect with your partner, take the pressure off and re-evaluate your plan for when you are ready to move forward with treatment again.

Whilst you're going through cycle after cycle it's important to set time aside for yourselves to do something you enjoy without thinking about the baby stuff. You will probably find you don't have much money if you're doing fertility treatment but just watching a movie together or going for a walk, anything that doesn't involve baby making talk.

Most importantly don't stop living which is totally different to just existing and going through the motions.

I remember a few times not going out because I didn't want to drink as it was around my fertile time. However, most of the time I never fell pregnant so I should have just gone out, relaxed and enjoyed myself. This is what I mean by don't stop living!

I can't imagine what it would be like to not get my baby at the end of all the stress and emotion that is fertility treatment but I know that sometimes this is the case and boy does my heart go out to those couples.

I can't say what these couples should do or how they must be feeling but in these cases I guess it would be even more important not to lose sight of yourself and your partner, to keep your social life going and to have other interests.

This is also something you should discuss before embarking on this process. 'What will we do if we don't fall pregnant?'

I know for myself there was one stage in particular during this process when I was thinking I didn't know how much longer I could keep going. It was all just getting too hard but I did already have my daughter so I'm sure I could have coped if I had made that decision to stop. If I hadn't already had a child it would have been extremely difficult to move on, especially seeing as my whole being had been stripped away, I wasn't working and didn't have much of a social life. It is so important to plan and discuss these things before you start.

Take your time looking for a specialist. If you're happy with them I believe it goes a long way to helping with this process. You will need someone that you are completely comfortable with and who you trust as you will be in some compromising positions at your most vulnerable times with this person.

More importantly meet the nurses at the office. You will have more contact with them than your doctor. They are the ones who will be phoning you about everything throughout your cycles, they perform your ultrasounds and if you choose IUI they will also perform your inseminations. At the end of your cycles they will give you either the good news that you are pregnant or the bad news that you need to begin treatment all over again. If you have questions or queries between appointments with your doctor they are your contact people and are therefore very important during this process.

Fertility treatment is a very full on process and you need to go into it with your eyes wide open.

4.
IVF – A Life Spent Waiting

People often talk about the dreaded two week wait when you're trying to conceive. This is the time from when you have ovulated till the time you either get your period or you are in fact pregnant. It is this period of time that seems to drag on forever.

Unfortunately when you're doing fertility treatment there are many other steps in the month that also feel like this and it feels like you spend your life constantly waiting.

So you find out you have your period again. Complete devastation follows and that hole in your heart seems to get a little bit bigger. You then have to wait for your period to stop which feels like the longest period anyone in the world has ever had.

You then wait to start the blood tests and then the wait to start the endless injections.

Now it's the wait for your eggs to become big enough. You have an internal ultrasound to see if the eggs are ready but sometimes they're not so you wait yet again.

You're finally ready to have your eggs collected so you wait around to go into theatre.

After that you wait to see if the embryos the lab has created make it to the following day, then the next day. Sometimes it can be up to five days after your egg collection before they phone and say it's time.

Yippee, finally embryo transfer time so you wait to go into theatre again and have that ever so personal transfer then you wait to see if the embryo has implanted.

Waiting, waiting, waiting, if you're lucky you hit the jackpot but it you're not it just starts all over again. You feel like your life is forever on hold.

I am not surprised that some marriages don't survive, it is a tough and sometimes very long road.

You need to have a very understanding partner to put up with the mood swings from all the different drugs you are injecting and the emotions. He needs to realize that you have no control over the way you are acting or feeling and that it is just so tough the endless poking, prodding and invading of a woman's body.

5.
The Needles

The injections, where do I begin?

You need to self-inject needles with both IUI and IVF so I was doing it for a long time and I'm not going to lie, it sucked. I can only tell you from what my experience was, which may of course be different from others. Some women may have very little side effects.

I wasn't particularly worried or feeling daunted by the prospect of having to inject myself because needles don't bother me. However it was at times painful and you begin to feel like a pin cushion.

There are three types of injections I had to take during a cycle and some hurt more than others. Sometimes they go in your thigh and sometimes in your stomach.

When I first started they didn't seem too bad but after a while they started hurting a little more and sometimes I would get a red tender lump, a rash or both.

I even started to tense up when I had to go for my blood tests which I had never had a problem with before so it does start to affect you if not at the beginning, eventually.

The injections definitely turned me into someone at times I didn't recognize and certainly didn't like. I could be happy one minute and fly off the handle about the smallest of things the next. It felt like I wasn't me anymore so I can only imagine how hard that was for my husband and daughter.

I would often think to myself that this is not who my husband chose to marry and why was my daughter having to put up with all of my grumpiness when she was such a good girl. That's when you get major feelings of guilt but as much as you try you cannot control how you act and how you feel.

Some of the injections you have to take actually contain the pregnancy hormone (you take these towards the end of your cycle) so they can bring on pregnancy symptoms even if you're not pregnant.

It was silly the amount of times I had convinced myself I was pregnant because I was having so many of the pregnancy symptoms. Then I would think how incredibly stupid I was to let myself go there yet again to then have that devastating blow at the end of the month when I would find out that of course I wasn't pregnant.

I found those injections extremely cruel.

6.

Emotions

Oh my god, you name any emotion and you will probably experience it at some stage. Some are good, but some are really bad and can hit you when you least expect them.

Pain – both physical and mental. I found I could cope much easier with the physical pain rather than the mental. The emotional pain is very hard to deal with.

Scared – the fear of the unknown and that even though you're doing everything you possibly can it's still out of your hands.

Lonely – sometimes it feels like you're completely on your own and that no one knows what you are going through. Even though your partner is traveling the journey with you it's still not the same.

Stress – the whole process brings with it a lot of stress and pressure and it can come from a few different areas. Number one, the procedures not working which can lead to problems in your relationship. Number two, the hormones in the injections. Number three, struggling financially and finally the pressure on the guys to perform at a moment's notice.

I think of all the times my husband had to produce a sperm sample on the spot with so much pressure and he's just done what he had to do.

I can't imagine the pressure of having to see your partner take injection after injection, having her personality stripped bare and then knowing that unless you produce the goods she would have done all of that for nothing.

Anger, bitterness and frustration – why isn't this working when it comes so easily to others?

Inadequate and failure – I always felt like this because as a woman this is what your body is meant to do. It is supposed to be the most natural thing in the world.

Sad and depressed – sometimes you get just plain and simple sad about the whole situation you have found yourself in and you can get quite depressed at times.

Humour – some of the things you need to do will be embarrassing and you just have to find humour in these situations. We had a few fits of laughter which usually occurred during sperm samples.

Looking back there was the time hubby had to do a sample in a room which was off to the side of the waiting room. However everyone in the waiting room could see you going in and of course they all knew what went on in there. The room was so tiny with a little single bed in the corner and some adult magazines. It felt like we were kids on a school camp doing something naughty.

Another time it was like a fancy hotel room. Very spacious with a leather couch, fridge, TV with DVD and of course adult movies.

Then one day because it was so early in the morning no hospitals were open to do the sample so hubby had to do it in the doctor's office. Not exactly the best place but my hubby was a real trooper.

Pure joy and happiness – if you're lucky enough to become pregnant after waiting for so long then there really is nothing like finding out that your miracle has happened.

There are many more emotions and feelings you will go through and it's so important to keep communicating with your partner about them. If you can be open and honest about your emotions and feelings then they might be able to at least see where the snappiness or moodiness is coming from instead of just thinking they've done something wrong. Sometimes we have to spell it out for our men!

I found that keeping a journal or just writing down a few things helped me with what I was feeling and dealing with the frustration.

If you can't talk to someone about your feelings you need to at least write them down. I wish I had done that the whole way through. I only began noting things down strangely enough the cycle that I fell pregnant which then resulted in a miscarriage.

It seems someone up above must have been telling me things were about to get worse and I would need a way of coping.

7.
Pet Peeves

In all fairness some of the things that people have said to me in the past were said without knowing that we were having so much trouble conceiving which is probably why you shouldn't keep it a secret. You may be able to save yourself from some very hurtful comments.

In saying that for some people it doesn't matter if they know or not, some just have no filter on their mouth or they're missing a sensitivity chip.

Some of my personal favourites are:

'Oh my husband only has to look at me and I'm pregnant'.

'Don't you know how to do it properly yet? Do you want me to show you?'

'What have you got dry ball?'

The amount of times we were asked that dreaded question 'When are you going to have a baby" was unbelievable but then it was probably worse when people stopped asking the question because then you feel like a complete failure especially if others have given up.

You can feel like the losers who can't have kids especially in my family where fertility seems to be anything but a problem which brings me to my next point – accidents!

I detest the word accident when describing how someone becomes pregnant. Hearing that makes you feel even more worthless because you are trying absolutely everything to get pregnant and they can accidentally without a thought or care in the world do what you desperately want to do yourself.

Babies are precious miracles to couples who have trouble conceiving, they are not accidents.

I cringe when I hear couples whining that they wanted a boy but had a girl or they 'really' hope they get a certain sex. This is so frustrating to hear because for many of us we would take any baby, boy or girl it wouldn't matter just as long as we get one precious baby.

Some other words of wisdom:

'Take a holiday'.

'Just relax and don't think about it. You know that some people who adopt fall pregnant naturally straight after because they stop thinking about it'.

Well here's some news, I tried all of that and more.

I started using Ovulation Predictor Kits and I would also check my cervical mucus and feel my cervix to find out when it was the most fertile time.

When that didn't work we tried doing the deed every second day just so we knew that there would always be swimmers in there for the right day. I would also lay down with my legs in the air for ages after doing the deed so that no little swimmers would escape.

You name it I probably tried it and nothing worked.

There is also this strange phenomenon when you are trying to conceive. Everyone around you, your family and friends are all falling pregnant and everywhere you go you will see pregnant bellies or newborn babies.

It can be really hard when you find out that yet another relative or friend is pregnant, it feels like a kick to the stomach every time. Don't get me wrong I was always genuinely happy for others but I would be jealous and really sad at the same time because I just wished it was happening to me.

Having trouble conceiving can be so absolutely devastating and sole destroying that unless you have walked in the same shoes as me I could never make anyone really understand what it has been like. I never wanted to be wrapped in cotton wool or have people feel sorry for me and have to watch what they said, just a bit of sensitivity would have been nice.

8.
Being Positive

So many people tell you to just think positive and it will happen. While it doesn't always work I do think being positive and having a laugh helps to some degree even if it's just for your own state of mind.

When we did our first IUI cycle with our first child after two years of trying the nurse came in to do the insemination and she said 'Now this doesn't always work so don't feel too bad if it doesn't happen'. So of course I went in thinking positive but after hearing that I was a bit down.

I went straight home to put my feet up for the rest of the day. I refused to go to the toilet for hours after just in case I lost some of those precious swimmers and thought about the nurse's comment for the rest of the day. That was not a successful cycle.

For the second IUI I had a different nurse and she had a really happy, sunny personality. Her words to me were 'Wow we have millions and millions of healthy sperm here, surely one is going to make it'. I was in a happier and more positive mood because of her words and off I went straight to work after the insemination which kept me busy for the rest of the day. I also went to the toilet as soon as I got to work. That turned out to be the cycle that produced our first baby.

It just goes to prove that it doesn't matter what you do it's either going to happen or it isn't so my advice is to just keeping going about your normal everyday lives.

When I had my embryo transfer for our second child I remember saying to my doctor about how I thought I was literally going to burst as I really needed to go to the toilet (you need to have a full bladder for a transfer). Of course he then made some teasing comment to which I replied something along the lines of 'I wouldn't be teasing me when I'm really not exaggerating and your about to have your head down there'. Everyone had a laugh and it was a really relaxed atmosphere considering I had my legs up in the air with five other people standing around watching.

The doctor also pointed out that the embryo was really well placed and had already started to hatch so it was a very positive environment and I did fall pregnant that cycle.

This is why it's so important to feel comfortable and happy with your doctor and his staff.

9.
Miscarriage

Miscarriage, it's a mysterious dark word that no one wants to talk about except for the ones that have experienced it. We do want to talk about the baby who was already growing in our belly. It would be nice for others to at least acknowledge that there was a baby and to try to understand why we are feeling so devastated.

We're not after some infinite wisdom or for you to have all the answers. Just say 'I'm sorry for your loss' or 'I'm really sorry this has happened, if you ever need to talk I'm here to listen'. It's better to say something like that than say nothing at all. At the very least acknowledge it has happened.

When people don't say anything it feels like they either don't care or they have already forgotten. That is probably not what they are thinking or feeling but they obviously don't know what to say or they don't want to bring it up for fear of upsetting you.

The thing is when this happens you are thinking about it every minute of the day anyway so someone saying something about it is not going to upset you, you're already upset. It can feel like the end of the world and you're not thinking clearly or even rationally so you tend to take things that are said or not said very emotionally and to heart.

The one thing I hated being told was that there must have been something wrong with it. For a start it's not an it, he or she was our much wanted baby and secondly we have just had our hearts completely shattered by this loss and then it's like kicking the boot in to hear there was probably something wrong with our baby. Just say you're sorry and leave it at that, it's not that hard surely?

It also doesn't matter if you are five weeks pregnant or five months pregnant it's still a loss at any stage and you need to grieve.

When I told people I was seven weeks pregnant it felt as though they were thinking that it wasn't long enough to be so invested and upset about but for me it was. I had known for three weeks that our miracle was growing inside which was something we wanted so desperately and had done so much to achieve. My body was already changing and more importantly I had a connection with my baby. We already had hopes and dreams for him or her.

I remember how it started. It was a Friday and I was at work when I had felt a few niggling pains but I had those all throughout my first pregnancy so I didn't think much about it.

However the next morning after I'd been to the toilet I noticed some spots of blood. As soon as I saw it I felt this awful feeling deep down in my soul and my heart started pounding. I kept thinking surely life couldn't be this cruel to finally be pregnant after all we'd been through and to be on such a major high for three weeks and then to lose the baby? No, that couldn't happen.

I phoned the doctor's office but it was a Saturday so they couldn't see me but I spoke to a nurse who told me that some women have bleeding and everything turns out fine with the baby, however it could also mean I was having a miscarriage. I was told I had to wait and see. Well IVF is the world of waiting so we had no choice but to wait.

I'll never forget the next morning passing what was obviously our precious and much loved baby. It was like someone had kicked me in the stomach, instant pain and heartache. I cried buckets of tears over the next few days and even when I really tried to force myself to stop they just kept coming until eventually I ran out of tears.

I had always felt so sorry for women who had been through a miscarriage but had never thought it would happen to me. Now I was living it and I truly understood how incredibly awful it was. No one can really know unless they have experienced it.

A dark cloud hung over me for a long time even though I still had so much in my life to be thankful for. I even had someone tell me that maybe I should forget about having another baby as maybe it's not meant to be and to be thankful that I had my daughter. Excuse me? Don't dare tell me that I'm not grateful or thankful for my daughter and if I took that advice of maybe it's not meant to be I wouldn't even have her because she was conceived through assisted conception. No I wasn't going to accept that this was how it was meant to be, I was so insulted and very hurt.

Such comments feel so insensitive at a time when you feel so vulnerable, isolated and you know they don't have a clue to what you are going through.

10.

How to Deal with Miscarriage

I don't think there is any particular way to deal with a miscarriage. It can be many different things for different people and time.

Looking back now I definitely should have seen someone to talk to about our loss. I always felt like no one around me wanted to talk about it so most of the time I just put a smile on my face and pretended I was okay when in fact I was falling to pieces on the inside.

Talking to someone who is not personally involved and who is a professional would have been the way to go. My clinic had someone you could see but I'm not sure why I didn't go. I guess I thought I could handle it on my own.

You need time to deal with grief and distraction is a wonderful thing for a little while but the issue will always be there so you still need to actually deal with your loss instead of hiding it away or pretending everything is fine.

Crying is a good thing. I used to think I was weak for crying and would try not to but it's just a way of your body dealing with what has happened. Never fight with your feelings, just go with them.

Finding someone who has been through the same thing is great because you can talk to them freely and honestly knowing that they understand how you feel and you don't feel quite so alone.

I was very surprised to find out how many others have had miscarriages and yet if I hadn't mentioned mine I would never have known. I'm not sure why women don't talk about miscarriage especially seeing as we seem to talk about every other subject.

I often wonder if there is a little bit of blame on our part thinking maybe we did something to cause the miscarriage or maybe we don't want to break down and show just how vulnerable we can be. It is such a shame that women don't discuss it as this is when we need the comfort from others the most.

I did eventually find a way that really did help, having a keepsake box. I bought a pretty box and inside I put a baby rug, an angel teddy, my pregnancy test, a note to our baby and a few other sentimental things. I keep it in a room where we spend a lot of time and it's just a way of remembering and acknowledging our angel baby.

11.
Looking Back

We have just arrived home after our insemination and now all we can do is hope and pray and hope and pray some more that this time it will work and we will get our baby.

It will be torture having to wait two weeks to find out if indeed we are pregnant. This process had been so hard emotionally but we know it will all be worth it in the end. To hold your newborn baby in your arms for the first time is absolute magic. Time stands still as you get lost in that precious moment.

This is just one of the reasons we would like to have another child. That and the amazement in a baby or child's eyes as they see and learn different things for the first time. It's priceless.

You see the world in a whole new way, sometimes for the better and sometimes for the worst. You soon realize when you have a baby to be responsible for that the world can be a scary place and you just want to protect them from everything.

To have a baby growing in your belly is such a privilege and brings so much joy and hope for the future. What an amazing and special time in your life.

We hope that in two weeks' time we can say with pride and

happiness that we are expecting and that will mark a whole new chapter in our lives.

We have just had our phone call to give us our results and it's so frustrating because they can't actually tell us either way if we are pregnant or not. Apparently HCG levels should be 30 or more if you are pregnant and mine are only 23 so they just don't know. I have to have yet another blood test on Monday to give us more news. Another four days of agonizing, waiting and wondering.

Wow we can't believe it. I phoned the nurse for our results and she said 'Congratulations' so we are finally pregnant. We are just so thrilled and can't seem to wipe the smiles off our faces. It's still a little hard to believe after we have wanted you so badly. I can't wait to hold you in my arms. When I told mum and dad they were so excited but also very relieved for us. I can't wait to have you grow bigger and bigger in my belly.

I am sitting here writing this with my heart broken in two and tears streaming down my face. We have lost you and I am completely and utterly shattered. My heart is so heavy with all the dreams and hopes we had of you that are now gone. I only had you in my belly for a short time but you were already such a part of me and I loved you so very much.

So we've just finished my fertile week and we have done the best we can. We figured if we were ever going to fall pregnant on our own then this month would be our best shot.

It's been three weeks since we lost our bub and although we will never forget we think the best way to move on is to try and fall pregnant as soon as possible so we can have something positive to focus on instead of this heartache. I have heard people say there's a good chance of conceiving just after you've been pregnant because the 'oven's still warm' so we gave it our best effort. Now it's totally out of our hands and we just need to wait and see.

It's probably not likely to happen for us but you just never know, sometimes miracles do happen. It would be so nice to know that we did it ourselves and that I didn't have to go back to taking injections, having blood tests and all the rest that comes with it. It's just so full on and exhausting especially emotionally. We have also looked into IVF but it's quite expensive. I guess you're paying for a greater chance of success, 40-50% instead of the 15-20% we are getting.

I often wonder what it's like for the majority of couples who just one day decide to try for a baby. Then they try and a couple of months later they are pregnant without a moment's thought. No one telling them when they are allowed to do the deed or how often they need to do it, no worrying about the expense of treatment, the risk of having multiples and the list goes on.

We are just hoping and praying that we get our little miracle.

Well unfortunately we didn't get the miracle we wanted. It wasn't really much of a surprise, I mean we've been let down so many times now that you tend to expect it. It's also easier to expect a bad outcome rather than being really positive and then having that huge let down when you find out it hasn't worked yet again and you feel as though your heart has been broken a little bit more.

We are trying to look forward now to the next month when we start fertility treatment again. At least doing that we know we have the best possible chance of making our baby. I hate the thought of having to inject myself with the needles again but I know that's what I have to do to achieve our dream, so let us begin.

So I had my ultrasound today which has left me yet again devastated. They found that I had three eggs which means they have cancelled the rest of my cycle. They say the risk of twins or triplets is too high and that we shouldn't try it ourselves naturally either. I still need to have two more injections and then my trigger shot to release the eggs and that is just plain cruel.

It's so tempting to try and conceive by ourselves because there are three good eggs in there that will just go to waste otherwise. It would be such a great chance to fall pregnant with three eggs but then you can just imagine if all three fertilized.

I still can't believe how this can happen especially as I was taking the same amount of drugs as I always have but I managed to produce three eggs instead of the usual one or two.

I'm so upset because it's another month of not fulfilling our dreams and we didn't even get to give it a try but yet I still had to go through all the injections and moods for nothing.

Worse still I had a huge meltdown at work. I had to go straight to work after my ultrasound and by the time I got there I was so upset. I think because not many people know what's been going on it has meant I've had things bottled up for too long. I found I just couldn't hide my emotions anymore and it all began to spill out. The result was not pretty. My poor work colleague thought that someone had died.

When I could eventually talk without crying I explained what had been going on and that I had recently had a miscarriage. She then told me she had miscarried years ago so in the end it was quite therapeutic talking to her. However it's starting to feel like it's never going to happen.

This week was also the time that we would have been three months pregnant and should have been telling everyone that we were having a bub but instead it's just a shit week of shattered dreams yet again.

Today I have started my injections again and then I find out another cousin is pregnant. I am really happy for them but the fact that it was an accident just really pisses me off.

When is it our turn? We are good people who work hard and do the right things in life and yet this is so damn difficult for us, but not others. Jealous? Yep guess I am.

So basically I feel like shit today and just want to go to bed and cry but of course that's not an option. I have to put on a happy face and pretend that everything is perfectly okay when in fact I feel like my whole world is falling apart.

Of course then I feel guilty thinking like that because I have a wonderful husband, daughter and a loving family so I should be grateful for that which obviously I am but there's just this empty feeling inside of the baby we lost and the one we are trying to create.

Why is life so hard sometimes? I want the chance to just fall pregnant and be able to enjoy my pregnancy without being totally stressed and exhausted by the time I eventually fall pregnant and then even more exhausted when the baby actually gets here. That's what happened the first time around after taking so long to fall pregnant and then being sick for the whole nine months.

I am already starting to think I'll just be so glad when we have another baby and then we never have to worry about all this stuff again. As much as we might want more children we will never go through this again. It is too much pain to go through month after month, disappointment after disappointment.

We had our insemination yesterday which was quite exciting because of the fact that we haven't been able to try for the last few months and doing this gives us such a better chance of falling pregnant. We know there are two eggs in there with millions and millions of sperm and we only need one little swimmer to get the job done so we are feeling really positive.

I have also been feeling much calmer than I normally am which is different. Usually I can't sleep the night before my ultrasound or insemination but I did this time so fingers crossed that it's a good sign. I'm sure the next two weeks are going to drag by so slowly but if we fall pregnant it will be worth the wait.

Please let this be our time for a bubby, we have been extremely patient and have gone through so much. It's totally amazing to think that as I write this we could indeed have a sperm fertilizing one of my eggs.

Well it's been one week and two days since our insemination and while it has gone quick in some ways, in others it's going so slow. Night time is worse because you actually get a chance to really sit down and think about things. I guess we're impatient and just want to know either way.

Today I had some time where I felt really tired and if I'd closed my eyes I think I would have fallen asleep which is very unusual for me and I've been really tired quite early in the evenings as well. This happened the last time I was pregnant so I am very hopeful. I just hope it's not those injections playing a cruel trick on me as that has happened many times before with some of the symptoms I have had.

I've also been having days where I just feel different. I feel at times like my heart is racing and that I get out of breath easily which is not normal either.

I only have one more injection to go tomorrow and then my final blood test on Tuesday so fingers, toes, everything crossed.

I'm so upset about not being pregnant that I don't even have anything to say. I don't know how much more of this I can take.

Starting injections today and I have promised myself that this month no matter how many pregnancy symptoms I have or how pregnant I feel I am going to deny it and pretend it's not happening. It is too damn hard to go through that disappointment. I have definitely learnt my lesson.

Well not pregnant again. Even though I didn't get my hopes up too high this time it still hurt like hell.

Wow excited much I'm about to start my first IVF cycle. I am starting on 125 units of puregon instead of the usual 25/50 units doing IUI so I'm wondering how my body will react with much more of the drug than normal.

Well the two injections I have had every day for the last six days are taking a toll. Feeling like a pin cushion, ouch.

Today I had my ultrasound because my eggs have grown really quickly and I have 21! Nice to know all the extra units of purogen were worth it.

Today is Friday and it's egg collection day, finally. The doctor took out eleven eggs however one wasn't mature enough so ten were collected.

Today, day one after collection the lab phoned to say that all ten eggs had fertilized woohoo!

Today is day three after collection and all ten are still going strong. I am starting to feel really excited but trying not to get too ahead of myself as I know there is still quite a way to go.

Today is Wednesday day five. Six of them have all gone to blastocyst stage so five have been frozen and I am booked in today to have one transferred.

I am feeling very anxious as I am waiting to go into theatre because I have a stupid cold and don't feel so great which is not how I would like to be feeling on such an important day. I'm hoping this cold will not have a negative effect on my transfer.

My doctor told me during my transfer that the blastocyst had already started hatching which is apparently good because as soon as it hatches it can implant. The staff in the lab also told us that all six blastocysts look textbook perfect so things are looking super fantastic and seeming a little too good to be true.

Tonight I am lying in bed and I feel strong cramping, please let this be implantation cramping.

Today is the day after my transfer. I have sore and bigger breasts already and I am very tired but these are also symptoms of the gel I have to use so it's probably just that.

By the way this gel is so gross and messy, having to insert it is not the best either but I know it's important. How many more to go? Too many to count, yuck.

The lab phoned today about our four remaining embryos. Three hadn't gone any further past day three and the other reached blastocyst stage but didn't look great so they have disposed of those which sounds awful but trying to think of all the positive things at the moment.

I am a couple of days post transfer and my tummy is quite bloated. You are bloated during IVF treatment anyway but they say if you become pregnant you will become even more bloated, trying not to get my hopes up too much. The veins on my boobs are also more noticeable (like a road map), I am extremely fatigued and even fell asleep during the day which only ever happens when I'm pregnant. I can smell perfume and deodorant on everybody and it's awful. I also had a chocolate donut which I normally love but it didn't taste too good.

I remember being pregnant with Jenna and my sense of smell was absolutely amazing. I could smell every little smell and

I went off most foods but I'm still trying to keep a lid on my excitement.

Well today is Monday and the nurse phoned to say that we are in fact finally pregnant. We are so thrilled and excited there are just no words.

It was really strange but about half an hour before I received the phone call from the nurse Jenna was sitting on the couch next to me when she started rubbing and touching my belly. I asked her why she was doing that and she said 'Because I love your tummy and you've got a bubby in there'. Dad was with us at the time but we didn't think too much of it until later when I took the phone call. Of course I told Jenna straight away and then rushed to Derren's work to tell him.

The news has sunk in a little and I feel so happy but very, very nervous and cautious. Please baby stick tight.

12.
Lessons I've Learnt

This IVF roller coaster ride has taught me many things.

Love is worth fighting for – no matter how stressful and hard the road is the love between you and your partner is worth every bit of suffering to come through to the rainbow at the end of the ride. I know not everyone makes it to the rainbow but I have learnt things about my husband and seen different sides of him that I probably wouldn't have if we hadn't gone through this.

He has been wonderful through this whole process and has had the patience of a saint to put up with all the drama that is assisted conception and has never once blamed me.

Your baby will be worth it – with everything bad that may have happened along the way when you look into that precious face and see life through a child's eyes bad memories are not forgotten but they can be pushed a little further to the back of your mind and your focus is directly on this tiny little soul.

Support from your family and friends will be tested – you will learn at the end of your journey who your real friends are and the family members you can count on.

There will be particular people who you know don't want to listen or they are uncomfortable talking about situations and there will be some real gems who try their best to understand.

The good friends are not always the ones constantly asking you about your cycles. They are the ones who treat you like the same person you were before trying to conceive and you will just know you can talk to them about anything if you need to.

Some people will ask you how you're going but you can tell they are not being genuine and are just being nosy.

Try not to judge others – you soon learn not to sweat the small stuff and before trying to conceive I was quite judgemental of others in normal everyday life.

When I was diagnosed with melanoma if I ever heard people complaining about petty things I would think 'My god imagine if you really had something to complain about, you would never cope! If only that was all I had to worry about.' However since trying to conceive my views have definitely changed.

I was secretive about the trouble we were having conceiving our first child so when I would see people in a bad mood instead of criticizing them I'd think 'Well they might be going through a really rough time at the moment'.

No one knows what really goes on in somebody else's life and what people choose to stress or moan about, even if it doesn't seem like much to you is obviously a crisis to them in their life so I am more empathetic and easy going in that regard.

What doesn't kill you makes you stronger - there is also a saying that you only get sent what you can cope with. Well I'd say this may or may not be true but I'm telling whoever is upstairs that I'm strong enough now thank you very much. My coping skills have well and truly been tested so that's enough now.

You certainly don't know how strong you can be or need to be until these things are sent to test you. I feel now having gone through all of this that no matter what happens in the future we can get through anything. It may be a fight or you may even have to drag or crawl your way through but you can make it.

13.
Ending

I am strong, determined and I have fought my hardest to have my babies.

I am totally in awe of anyone out there traveling the same road that may not yet have achieved their dream or may never achieve it. I wish that wasn't the case as everyone should have the chance to be a parent.

I hope that couples reading this can somehow be a little more prepared for what they are about to embark on or if you know someone going through this emotional time then maybe you can try to understand them a little more or be more of a shoulder to lean on.

To those of you who are on this journey already and are waiting for their miracle I send you millions and millions of baby dust and pray that it works out for you. If it doesn't I hope you can find a way to live your lives without the huge sadness of that one missing piece of your heart weighing you down.

Knowing what I know now and after being through some very difficult times I would go through all of it again in an instant. Holding your baby in your arms for the first time is worth every bit of pain, sadness and heartache.

The only thing I would change is being much more informed, therefore more prepared and I would have a plan for every step of the way.